Fight Stress and Live!

Fight Stress & *Live!*

5 Simple Commitments That Can Save Your Life

GENETTE HOWARD

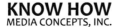
KNOW HOW
MEDIA CONCEPTS, INC.

Know How Media Concepts, Inc.
P.O. Box 3682
Fayetteville, AR 72702
479-251-7327

Published by: Know How Media Concepts, Inc. 7/20/2012

ISBN: 978-0-9849720-0-5 (soft cover)

CONTENTS

DEDICATION

This book is dedicated to my husband, Dexter Howard, who lives and loves courageously as the only man in a house filled with women.

"But the tongue of the wise promotes health."
                                        Proverbs 12:18

ACKNOWLEDGMENTS

The words in this book are from a heart that has been refined through the fires of life. My journey has been difficult since day one. Nothing has come easy for me. It is only by the grace of God and the wisdom of His Word that I am alive, healthy and happy today. Now my passion is to encourage and equip others to face life's challenges head on with wisdom, knowledge, and faith in the living God.

There are no words to express my love and appreciation for my husband, Pastor Dexter Howard and our six daughters: Alexa, Bethany, Celeste, Destiny, Eden and Faith. When I was voted "most likely to succeed" in high school, I never imagined that my success would consist of birthing this special family. Now I can't imagine anything better. I wouldn't change a thing. I hope I make you proud as I tell our story.

To my mother and father, Mr. and Mrs. Evans Seawood, Jr. Thank you for the exceptional home training, work ethic, discipline, and good common sense you instilled in me. They are priceless treasures in my heart.

To my mother-in-love, Maxine Webb. Thank you for sharing the load of the Howard family. I know how heavy we can be.

To my sisters, Angela and Evease; and my brothers, Greg, Rodney, and Chris. We are a testament to the faithfulness of Almighty God. If we can make it anybody can.

To my Restoration Church family, this includes my exceptional staff and ministry team. I believe deeply in spiritual family and I'm grateful to have you in my life. I love you all.

Last but never least, to the treasure of my universe, Jesus Christ. You are everything.

FOREWORD

Stress has become such a common word in our vocabulary that we are desensitized to its real and deadly impact. For 27 years I have practiced Internal Medicine, and have witnessed the effects of stress as it gradually but overwhelmingly undermined the physical and mental health of hundreds of patients. Though most of them worried more about dying from cancer or having a heart attack, they failed to acknowledge the major instigator of both of these diseases—CHRONIC STRESS.

For this reason, I write the foreword for this book. I am grateful that my dear friend, (Pastor) Genette Howard, has joined our fight against stress. The information contained in the following pages is simple, practical, and powerful. It will help every person who is ready to take action to sustain a longer and stronger life.

Stress is the God-given physiologic and biochemical RESPONSE of our bodies when facing difficult circumstances. Our adrenal glands release a hormone called cortisol as a response to stressors. Cortisol can be a lifesaver. For instance, when we are in danger and need to respond quickly, cortisol levels rise rapidly to give us the strength and energy we need to react. This hormonal surge is what causes a mom to lift a heavy object off her child or a passer-by to pull someone out of a burning car.

The adrenal glands release the amount of cortisol perceived necessary to handle the situation. It registers your response to the circumstance and reacts accordingly with the level of hormone needed. The problem with cortisol is too much of it can have deadly implications over time. The body was never intended to be in a constant state of emergency. Continual high levels of cortisol in the body can exhaust the adrenal glands and have disastrous effects if not checked.

> *The body was never intended to be in a constant state of emergency.*

Many of us think that the stressors are the real problem; but we are wrong. What makes the stress deadly is the way we handle it. It is really the way we perceive and react to difficult circumstances that determines how the body is affected. Research shows that most of us are not handling our over-committed, strenuous lifestyle well.

According to the Centers for Disease Control and Prevention, up to 90% of the doctor visits in the USA and half the deaths to Americans under age 65 may be triggered by a stress-related illness.

Chronic stress has been implicated in heart, stomach and mental disorders, along with common headache, backache, high blood pressure and cholesterol. A 10 year study of medical students during stressful exam times, found decreased levels of the body's natural killer (immune) cells, which fight infection and keep cancer in check. The effects of stress are real and measurable; it is nothing to play with.

Three years ago when I closed a busy, thriving primary care practice, I estimate that the vast majority of the office visits were stress related. The number of patients requesting completion of FMLA (leave) forms because of the pressures of their workplace and its effect on their physical and mental health had risen significantly—from a request once every two or three months to once or twice a week. I was overwhelmed at the documentation employers required to substantiate an employee's need for a leave due to stress. Obviously company officials did not understand the very real physical detriments of an over-taxing work environment.

Not only were my patients stressed and sick, so was I. The pressures of being a business owner; listening to and encouraging patients all day long; business overhead and decreasing reimbursement from insurance companies, left me physically and emotionally wasted with severe hormonal imbalances and adrenal fatigue. It has been a three year journey of recovery through consistent and purposeful lifestyle changes, supplementation and yielding of every part of my life to God, that has gotten me this far.

I have watched Genette Howard over the past seven years in several capacities including mother, wife, Pastor and leader, and wondered in amazement how she so gracefully regained and maintained her footing and balance in life and ministry. God divinely connected us following her sixth pregnancy and delivery as she moved from one of the lowest places in her life emotionally and physically. While she tells people that I "saved her life" by supporting her hormones during that dark time, I now understand that the real healing came as a result of the Godly wisdom she shares in the pages of this powerful book.

The good news is stress need not damage your health. If you will read, understand and apply the five simple commitments that Pastor Genette has provided in the following pages, you can quickly be on the road to a healthier, happier life. More importantly, you will be positioned to carry out God's purpose for your life in a way that will bring great joy and life to many others!

In His Service,

Rita C. Rodgers-Stanley, M.D.

To women everywhere who are speed-racing through each day, running to get to the next place like your hair is on fire. Stop. Get still. Breathe and listen. Your real life is waiting.

INTRODUCTION

It all began one Friday afternoon after picking up five kids at four different schools. It was a rare weekend when my husband was home and there were no ballgames, practices, events or family obligations in the next 24 hours. Every part of me was exhausted—my mind, body, and spirit. Even though it was a slow weekend in our house, I knew it would not be a quiet one. Not with six children on the premises. The prospect of rest for me was still slim and none.

I sat down beside my husband on the sofa and said, "I am so exhausted. I should go to a hotel and rest."

His response shocked me. "Yes, you should do that. Nothing's happening and I can hang out with the kids. Go ahead. We'll be fine," he said matter-of-factly as he began to flip channels on the TV.

I thought to myself, "Huh?" I really had no intention of going anywhere. I love my home and cherish being there. I guess I just wanted to talk about how tired I was so I could get some sympathy. But my husband is not the belly-aching kind. He is a solution-driven, man's man. I stated my problem and the answer, so to him it was a done deal. I was going to the hotel 10 minutes from my house to relax alone for 24 hours.

I slowly packed my little overnight bag with my cozy pjs, slippers, a change of clothes, and my journal to record some thoughts. I said good-bye to my daughters one by one; gave my husband a kiss as I took one last whiff of his cologne for my memory; then started my short journey to the hotel.

"Wow, you didn't come from very far," the desk clerk said as she observed my address at check in. I told her how many kids I have and that my husband sent me away for some rest.

I felt really silly standing there and expected her to look up at me suspiciously. Instead she responded in her excited southern drawl, "Wow, that's wonderful. You've got a great husband!"

The news seemed to spread among the staff that there was a tired mama of six daughters there for some peace and quiet. There weren't many guests that weekend so the cook and attendants happily catered to me. I walked around the hotel with my fuzzy slippers on and enjoyed the special treatment and friendly greetings, "Hey, how's your rest coming?" It was an unforgettable blessing.

When I got settled into my room for the evening and adjusted to the silence, God's voice began to speak to me. It was a warning about stress and how deadly it is. I was cautioned that the state I was in was not good and my days would be shortened if I didn't change my lifestyle. It was a very real encounter to me and I wept at the thought of leaving my family too soon. That was a significant turning point in my life. At that moment, stress became my enemy and I began to pursue a more peaceful way of life.

Stress is a slow killer. Women, especially, are under more of it than ever before. Those knots in your neck, shoulders, and back are filled with toxins. That burning sensation you feel in your stomach when you worry is a release of poisons into your system. Our mailboxes and TVs are filled with offers to help us reduce our weight and debt because everyone knows the danger of too much of those. But what about stress? It is actually the greatest detriment to our overall health and quality of life.

Stress is a slow killer. Women, especially, are under more of it than ever before.

Consider these amazing facts about today's woman:

- Women make up over 40% of the workforce.

- Women earn approximately 60% of all bachelor's and master's degrees.

- Women hold more management and supervisory positions than men.

- Women's pay is increasing faster than men's.

We are on the move like never before; however, our progress over the last 40 years has come with a cost.

Recent studies have discovered that women around the world are growing increasingly stressed, unhappy, and unhealthy. Here are some more startling facts:

- Over the last 40 years, women have become less happy than they were, and less happy than men.

- Women report being less satisfied with all aspects of life.

- Women's daily stress levels are higher now than they were 40 years ago, and adding more free time does little to lessen her feelings of stress.

- Women consume twice as much anti-depression and anti-anxiety medication as men.

I am all for progress, but I'm all-out AGAINST excessive, incessant stress and have declared war on it in my life. I want to live. To help you understand my passionate plea for you to join me in this fight against stress, let me tell you a little more about me.

I was an over-achieving workaholic. I have developed a pretty strong theory as to where that stemmed from, but that's another book. Being a mom of any number of children is demanding, but being the mom of six *girls* multiplies the effect because of the mega-details and drama that go along with the female persuasion. My personality is also predominately passive-aggressive, meaning I bottle my feelings in until I explode. For many years I was a walking internal *disaster* and I had more breakdowns than I can recall. I always managed to comeback, but of course, the cycle continued because my behavior pattern stayed the same. My motto was, "I don't sit down 'til I fall down." I just worked, worked, worked, until I couldn't stand up anymore, basically. I thought I was being a virtuous woman.

I was also success-driven at all costs. Although I am a fun-loving person, I denied myself opportunities to relax and have a good time with friends. I would go for weeks or months without talking to my sisters or girlfriends. I lost touch with many of them. I considered fun as a luxury I couldn't afford if I wanted to meet my goals. As a mom, most of the time my self-neglect was more about meeting the needs of others than it was about meeting a goal. As I look back that was a very sad time of my life.

When I turned 40, my body began to act weird. I had some in depth testing done and my doctor discovered that I had an intense case of adrenal fatigue, which is induced by incessant stress. If not addressed properly, fatigue of the adrenal glands can lead to multiple major illnesses and diseases. I was a ticking time-bomb. That was my first sign that something needed to change.

Then my menstrual cycle went AWOL. It just stopped at 41 years old. More testing revealed that I was in pre-mature menopause . . . at 41. One of the areas that I probably was a little prideful about was that I looked good for a mom of six—or at least that's what I was told constantly. "You have six children?" "You have teenagers? My, you look way too young." "Darling, you look wonderful." These were comments that I heard daily. I guess I believed them and assumed I was doing alright managing the madness that was my life.

But my bio-chemistry was telling a different story. According to my doctor, my hormonal levels read like a typical 51 year old, 10 years older than my actual age at the time. I may have looked like I was 10 years younger on the outside, but the lab results told the truth about my current physical state. I began to listen. Seriously. The culprit was non-stop stress, and much of it self-inflicted. If I was going to live *well*, I knew I had to master it in my life.

I must say that I do not think it is possible to live a stress-free life in today's world. Stress is simply the body's reaction to anything that throws off its delicate equilibrium. Life on earth among other imperfect human beings is stressful. The inevitable changes of life—births, deaths, successes, failures—are stressful. Relationships can be stressful. Environmental hazards, such as the weather, economy, traffic, and crime are stressful. Much of it is out of our control and it doesn't help that we get 24-hour news updates everywhere we turn. Because it is impossible not to encounter stressors in this life, it is vital that we find and use strategies to reduce it and its harmful effects.

In the following pages, I will share with you the five simple commitments I have made to myself to fight stress in my life. Each is a discovery I made as I actively sought knowledge and wisdom to live

In this modern, turbulent world, His Word is more relevant than ever.

a more peaceful life—even in the midst of chaos. My search for wisdom always begins in the Bible. I believe this Holy Book is the source of all eternal wisdom, knowledge, and understanding. In this modern, turbulent world, His Word is more relevant than ever. Naturally you will find many Biblical references in the pages to follow.

My desire is to live long and strong, so I can enjoy my family to the fullest and complete my God-given mission with physical strength and stamina. I have made the choice to fight stress and live. It is a daily challenge but I am committed.

Won't you join me? I invite you to make these five commitments your own, so you too can live a long, joyous life.

COMMITMENT ONE

I will enter my prayer closet daily.

"But you, when you pray, enter into your closet, and when you have shut your door, pray to your Father which is in secret."

Jesus Christ

Personally, this is the most important de-stressor in my life so I begin with this one: personal, private, intimate prayer. The picture that Jesus paints of prayer is one of privacy and deep intimacy. He not only teaches to find a secret place for prayer, a closet, but to make sure the door is closed so no one can see or hear you. Then he says that we should talk to our Father in heaven. Why is this so powerful for stress-relief and reduction? A bit more of my story may help explain.

I grew up in a troubled home. I saw and heard things that no child should. Like most children, I found a way to cope with a situation I couldn't control. I chose to suppress my emotions. I remember the day I decided to stop crying or talking about what was happening at home. It's like an epiphany came to me that tears and words don't change things, so why waste them? For the next 20 years or more, I got out of the "feelings" game, becoming a skilled suppressor-an expert at denying my true feelings about things. I mistakenly thought that I could shake anything off and handle everything on my own. I soon discovered that the pain didn't go away. Rather, I had closed my outlets, trapping the pain inside. You see, If we don't have a place for our emotional pain, worry, confusion and anxiety to go, it stays bottled on the inside of us. We become an internal cesspool. That's not just a metaphor but a real scientific fact. We have to have a place of release. This is the power of the prayer closet.

> *if we don't have a place for our emotional pain, worry, confusion and anxiety to go, it stays bottled on the inside of us. We become an internal cesspool.*

Talk It Out

The most important thing about prayer that Jesus taught us is that it is private and intimate conversation with our Father. It's as if God knows that we need to talk and the things we need to say are painful. Maybe even socially taboo. They are things we cannot, or should not, talk to any other human about. Still they have to be said. The negative emotions we store up on a daily basis have to have somewhere to go for our spiritual, mental, and physical health's sake.

Prayer is a privilege that we have to bring all of our humanity to God. Think about it. He's God. He knew us before we were born. He knows every detail about us, even the thoughts we are *going* to think. He knows what we will say before we utter it. He knows the decision we will make before we do. He is intimately acquainted with all of our ways, good and bad. He knows what we need before we ask. So why go through the trouble of talking to Him? It is because *you* need to talk. You need a place to go and a person to talk to where you can cast all of your cares without fear of ridicule, judgment, or shock. You need the release and the relief.

You may have a friend who is a great confidante that will hear you out. That is a great blessing, but they are a limited resource. Life is hard for everyone and they are carrying their own burdens. No human being can be the perfect support you need. Your welcome *can* wear out, even with a best friend or a spouse. Only the Eternal God is strong enough to carry all of our burdens.

In the prayer closet, you can let it all out. You can be transparent and genuine. There's no need for piety—we only need to be pious for people. There's no need for perfection—that's for people, too. We don't have to use impressive speech—that's for an audience. There's no need to fear doing or saying the wrong thing—you can't hurt God's feelings and you can't shock Him. Remember, He already knows it all. This is your opportunity to get the negativity out of you. Take it.

> *In the prayer closet, you can let it all out. You can be transparent and genuine.*

At first it may seem like you're talking to yourself because He lives in the unseen place. Our Father is invisible, but you must believe that He is there when you pray. Just use simple, child-like faith and take your audience with the God of the universe.

Cry It Out

Jesus wept. The greatest human that ever lived, the one who millions of people believe was God in the flesh, actually cried. The most notable occasion of him crying was recorded when his dear friend Lazarus died. As he approached the tomb of Lazarus with the intention of raising him up three days after his death, he looked around and saw the grief-stricken family. Although he knew their sorrow would turn to joy in just a few moments as he called Lazarus out of the grave; for some reason, he wept. Theologians still debate on exactly why he cried, but in my opinion, the reason doesn't matter nearly as much as the fact that he *did*. This great man was a human being and he responded to life through his emotions. If the occasion called for tears, he released them. He did not hold them back. I think this is the greatest revelation of the shortest verse in the Bible: Jesus wept.

Crying, in the proper context and timing, is a great practice for emotional health. Scientists have discovered that the chemical make-up of emotional tears is different than those produced from some other stimulus, like an onion, for instance. There is actually a chemical called leucine encephalin in tears that are released from joy, pain, anger, grief, or stress. This substance is a natural painkiller. I think that is amazing, because we all know that a good cry often makes us feel better. Yes, weeping can be a gift that gives us relief from the strain and pain of life. There is a definite catharsis—or purifying of the heart and mind of toxic feelings—that takes place when we shed tears.

There is a definite catharsis—or purifying of the heart and mind of toxic feelings—that takes place when we shed tears.

According to EveryDayHealth.com, one study analyzed 140 years of popular articles about crying and found that more than 9 in 10 found tears to be a good way to release pent-up feelings. An international sample of men and women from 30 countries found that most reported feeling relief after a good cry. And about 70 percent of therapists say they believe crying is good for their patients.

From my experience, the most healing cry is one that we release in the presence of unconditional love and support of another. That old saying about needing a shoulder to cry on has a lot of truth in it. After the tears are shed, a loved one can help with words of encouragement and positive reinforcements you need to move on.

This is the power of the prayer closet, as well. In the intimate place with your Father, you can cry it out if you need to. Sometimes you can't find words to express what you feel. That's when tears are necessary for your relief. Remember, God already knows everything. Just let the tears flow. Let them speak for you. He can interpret. Cry on His strong, everlasting arms.

Most importantly, stay in your place of prayer until the tears are dried and encouragement comes to your heart from above. God is a living being who loves you more than any other. He will speak words of hope and strength to you like no other person can.

Forgive—Let It Go

I've heard it said that unforgiveness is like drinking poison and expecting someone else to die. That would be ludicrous, wouldn't it? No matter how we want to justify it, unforgiveness is toxic to every part of our life: spiritual, mental, and physical. It is serious business and nothing to be toyed with.

Unforgiveness is holding on to hurt feelings, bitterness, and grudges caused by pain that was inflicted on you by another. It is also holding the person who hurt you in contempt, even to the point of being vengeful and wishing them harm. Oftentimes, you can be unforgiving of yourself for causing pain. Both states are equally dangerous. An unforgiving person will not only become an unhappy person, but also an unhealthy person, as the poison of bitterness seeps into every part of their life. The longer you hold onto offenses, the bigger they grow—like a tumor left untreated.

Research has found that unforgiveness is a leading cause of many physical ailments. Harboring bitterness and resentment raises blood pressure, depletes immune systems, stiffens joints, and makes you more easily depressed. It produces fatigue, lack of focus, and causes people to hold excess weight. All of these are major stressors on the physical body.

> *Harboring bitterness and resentment raises blood pressure, depletes immune systems, stiffens joints, and makes you more easily depressed.*

Unforgiveness also creates anger, mistrust, fear, and tension in relationships. Simply put, it blocks the way to hope, joy, peace, and love—all of the things that are vital to well-being and make life worth living. I hope you will agree that holding on to offenses is not an option if you want to live a long, healthy, and joyful life.

Life is tough and I believe you will not escape it without experiencing pain on some level. It is inevitable that every human being will be confronted with the decision to forgive or not to forgive and it won't be easy. I've often said that forgiveness is not natural; it's supernatural. It takes a power higher than our human ability to be able to release our pain and the source of it. We need help to forgive. Again, this is the wonder we find in the prayer closet.

Consider Jesus. He was betrayed and denied by his friends, unjustly tried and found guilty for crimes he had not done, and sentenced to die by crucifixion. Hanging on a cross between two notorious criminals, the innocent man cried out with his last breath, "Father, forgive them; for they know not what they do." He not only forgave his murderers, but he also prayed that God would forgive them. What an amazing demonstration of strength. More than any of his miraculous works, I believe that this final scene of his life as a man best proved that he indeed was the Son of God. He forgave. He let go of the greatest pain imaginable and prayed for his oppressors. Because he forgave, nothing could hold him down; not even death. His resurrection was imminent.

This is the kind of God you are meeting within your private place—a Father who not only asks you to forgive, but who has the power to forgive. The strength that you don't have as a hurting, wounded human, he *does* have and is waiting and willing to share his divine nature with you.

The prayer closet is also the place where you should first acknowledge your need to forgive and be forgiven. They are inextricably tied to each other, according to Scripture:

> *And whenever you stand praying, if you have anything against anyone, forgive him and let it drop (leave it, let it go), in order that your Father Who is in heaven may also forgive you your [own] failings and shortcomings and let them drop. But if you do not forgive, neither will your Father in heaven forgive your failings and shortcomings.*
> *Matthew 11:25, 26 Amplified*

Can you see how vital this personal, private time is with God for your well-being? Forgiveness—the ultimate stress relief—is waiting for you there.

Quick Tips

Here are some practical tips to help you as you make a commitment to a daily time of prayer:

- **Choose an intimate private place where you meet your Father.** This can be anywhere. Currently, my prayer closet is in my home office. In a room where I work that has a desk covered with contracts to negotiate and bills to pay; I carved out a special place in the corner so I can be one on one with my Father. It's nothing fancy, just a comfortable chair, a table and a lamp. It doesn't seem like I can find peace in a corner, but this one is different. It has a large window near and sunlight streams in from outside. I sit there and sip on my morning coffee for a few minutes as the warm rays soak into my skin. I look around my office at the pictures of loved ones and other beautiful things in the room. I'm inspired by beauty, so this little place is my own personal paradise.

  On the floor beneath my feet is a plush rug. I put it there to protect my knees from the hardwood, but even it has become special. Over the years I have soaked it with tears of sadness during bad times and ones of happiness when I'm overjoyed.

Whatever the case may be, I sit daily with my Father, letting it all go—problems, praise, and love. I'm thankful that currently I have nothing but gratitude and awe to give God for His faithfulness.

I've had all kinds of prayer closets over the years. I've somehow instinctively been drawn to a certain place in my home where I could be alone to pray. In one small house, it was the bathroom. In another, it was actually in an oversized closet. In the summer, I spend my early mornings on our back patio, listening to the birds sing while I talk to God. I've made prayer closets in my car and even on airplanes. In flight, I close my eyes and talk to my Father in my mind. He hears thoughts, too.

- **Begin by thanking your Father for all that He has done for you.** This is important. Even in a human relationship, it's appropriate to thank a person for the good things they've done before you begin pouring negative things on them. Approach your intimate prayer time with your Father this way. Gratitude is a wonderful practice to trade negative energy for positive energy. Your gratitude needs an outlet, too. Release thanksgiving.

> *Gratitude is a wonderful practice to trade negative energy for positive energy. Your gratitude needs an outlet, too. Release thanksgiving.*

Sometimes it's difficult to see the good things you have to be thankful for when you are encountering a hard situation. Pain can be blinding at times. Here are some guide posts to help you remember how much you have to be grateful for. Consider these things right now:

Are you alive? Yes you are!
Are you reasonably healthy?
Do you have the ability to think and reason on your own?
Do you have clean water, food, clothing, and shelter?
Do you have family and friends who love you?
Have you *ever* had anyone who loved you?
Have you overcome troubles in the past?
Has anyone been kind to you?

These are just a few questions to jog your memory of how much you have to be grateful for. Enter into your prayer time by thanking God first. It will change the atmosphere of your heart, mind, and even your prayer closet as you verbalize your gratitude to God.

- **Say what's in your heart. Say what you feel.** I know the great faith teachers say that we shouldn't live by our feelings, but by faith in God. That's true. But faith does not deny human feelings. Faith in God helps us move on regardless of our emotions. However, for our well-being we need an outlet for the things that daily store up in our heart and mind, especially negative ones. Talk to

God about your pain, confusion, worry or fears. Sometimes when we acknowledge and express the negative feelings, they lose their power over us. We are free to get up and move on.

Whatever you need to say; whatever it takes, get the emotions—good or bad—out of you. This is the wonderful opportunity you have in the prayer closet.

- **Forgive others and receive forgiveness.** Acknowledge any offenses you have with people. Talk to God about how their actions hurt you and then make a conscious decision to forgive them and let it go. Don't do this for them, do this for yourself. For your own well-being. Refuse to let one negative encounter inflict pain on you for the rest of your life. Free yourself from future harm by forgiving people quickly. If you need His help to do this, ask for it.

You may have heard people say that you can forgive but should never forget. I totally disagree. My personal practice is to forgive *and* to forget. I refuse to give the negativity anymore mental space. I purposely treat it like trash and throw it away. I firmly believe this is why I

> *My personal practice is to forgive and to forget. I refuse to give the negativity anymore mental space. I purposely treat it like trash and throw it away.*

have maintained a passion for my marriage, ministry, and life in general—the power of forgiving *and* forgetting.

It is equally important to receive forgiveness. In the prayer closet, you should confess your own faults and shortcomings. Lay it all out then receive God's wonderful forgiveness. His mercies are great and never run out. Walk in forgiveness.

I must say this . . .

Prayer is much more than an emotional outlet. Prayer is multi-faceted, spiritual communication, and it is unlimited in its power. Prayer literally has the power to change the world. Yet, in its simplest, most precious form, it is talking to your Father who knows and loves you perfectly. I encourage you to daily enter your prayer closet and cast the stresses of your life on Him, because He cares for you like no other.

> *"Cast all your anxiety on Him because He cares for you."*
>
> *I Peter 5:7*

> *"Come to me, all you who are weary and burdened, and I will give you rest."*
>
> *Matthew 11:28*

Right Now

What stresses do you need to cast on your Father?

What emotions do you need to release to Him?

Who do you need to forgive?

Do you need forgiveness? From what?

COMMITMENT TWO

I will find my Sabbath and keep it.

There are six days for work but the seventh day is Sabbath, pure rest, holy to God . . . Yes, because in six days God made the Heavens and the Earth and on the seventh day he stopped and took a long, deep breath. Exodus 11:15, 17 The Message Bible

God told Moses to command the Israelites to work six days and on the seventh day they were to do no labor. This day God called "Sabbath" and it was set apart as a time for rest only. This was a law and breaking it was a sin for the Israelites, also known as the Jews. On that day, everyone in the household—including servants and animals—was required to take a 24 hour break. God said if they obeyed Him by resting one day, they would be following His very own pattern for success. In six days He created the heavens and earth, and on the seventh day He took a long, deep breath.

The word "Sabbath" is originally "Shabbat" in the Hebrew language, which means "to cease", "to end", or "to rest". This commandment set the Jews apart from any other group of people. The idea of a weekly day of relaxation was never heard of before this time. The Greeks actually mocked the Jews for being lazy because of their commanded holiday every six days. However, God intended for this weekly sabbatical to set them high above any other group of people.

Life Works Best in Rhythm

We all know the importance of relaxation for the body and mind. I believe the significance of the Sabbath is in the *rhythm* of the rest that God commanded: work six days and cease from labor on the seventh day. It is the timing and recurrence of the reprieve that unlocks great productivity for those who keep it—every seventh day you stop, rest, and reflect. Think about it. Everything in nature works in a certain pattern that is highly predictable. We can forecast the time of sunrises and sunsets to the minute. Spring, summer, winter, and fall arrive at a designated moment every year. Animals instinctively know when to migrate to another climate each season. I could go on but I think you get the picture. All of creation is moving at a certain cadence that has been set. We can't hear the beat, but it's there. There is a dance of life that has been in motion at a specific tempo since the beginning. I believe this rhythm has been encoded in every living being, even humans, and life works best

> *When the rhythm is ignored, we suffer. We lose our beauty, majesty, and productivity. We diminish the image of God in us.*

when we move within the beat of our Creator. When the rhythm is ignored, we suffer. We lose our beauty, majesty, and productivity. We diminish the image of God in us.

Let's consider babies. They come into the world with a certain instinct of when it is time to eat, sleep and socialize. It soon manifests as a pretty predictable pattern. My whole world revolved around my children's eating and sleeping schedule when they were little. It took me awhile, but I finally discovered each of their patterns and kept it as consistent as possible. When I was able to work within the rhythm of their needs—providing meals, playtime and rest on schedule—the day went smoothly. They were happy and content. The days I could not were highly frustrating for us both. Cranky little ones are often trying to tell us that the cadence of their world has been violated. They were divinely designed to have their basic needs met consistently and predictably. This kind of environment helps them grow and perform at their best.

I believe the Sabbath reveals to us the pattern or rhythm of work and rest that all humans *need* to remain strong, creative, and productive. Work six days and chill out on the seventh day. It sounds simple, but in today's world it's not easily done. As we grow older, we tend to resist, even refuse, God's rhythm of life. Human beings are the only living creatures who have the liberty to do this, often to our demise.

> *The Sabbath reveals to us the pattern or rhythm of work and rest that all humans need to remain strong, creative, and productive. Work six days and chill out on the seventh day.*

My Southern Sabbath

Some religious faiths observe the Sabbath on Saturday, since our calendar lists it as the seventh day. But growing up in the Delta region of Arkansas, we considered Sunday as our holy day of the week. Whether you went to church or not, the whole culture acknowledged Sunday was the Lord's Day—a day for some to worship, but a day for all to rest. There really was not much else you could do because everything was closed, except hospitals and maybe a gas station here or there. In the Bible-belt south, we took this command to relax and reflect on the seventh day very seriously.

My family, in particular, didn't play when it came to obeying God's law of rest. Right now I can still smell the aroma of chicken frying, greens simmering, and cakes and biscuits baking in the oven on Saturday night. My mother or grandmother would be in the kitchen cooking the meal that we would eat the next day after church, as they hollered at us kids to get our clothes ironed for worship service and for the next week. Everyone scurried on Saturday getting shopping, cooking, and chores done because on Sunday there would be no stores opened and no labor. You see in my family, working on Sunday was a sin—a "get a whooping" sin, if you were caught.

One of my brothers would often try to sneak and iron his school clothes on Sunday night because he was hardheaded, mostly. But I also think he just didn't understand how ironing a pair of pants on Sunday was going to send him to the lake of fire. Sometimes he got away with it, but most times my mother would catch him.

"Boy, put that ironing board up! It's the Sabbath Day. Remember the Sabbath and keep it holy," she would say as she whopped him on the behind.

As a kid, Sunday was my favorite day of the week. I knew exactly what would happen. On the first and third Sunday, we only had Sunday School because our pastor was the leader of two different congregations. When he was at our church on the second and fourth weeks, we had "service" and he preached—the *same* sermon each week. The church members were my extended family and I loved chasing my friends and cousins down the steps of the country church and around the building after we were dismissed. I don't know why my mom would make us get all dressed up because we all looked like a mess after we finished playing tag and acting wild and crazy on the church yard.

We would say our goodbyes with hugs and kisses and head home to the delicious meal that was prepared on Saturday. Around my family's table, everyone would have to say a verse from the Bible before we could eat. That was even predictable, as everyone always said the same verse. My dad's was "None shall see God but the pure in heart." My oldest brother's was the shortest verse in the Bible: "Jesus wept". Mine was the longest of anyone's and I took great pride in repeating it weekly, "In my Father's house are many mansions. If it were not so I would not have told you. I go to prepare a place for you that where I am you may be also." My siblings thought I was a show-off but my dad was impressed every time.

After the weekly argument about who would wash dishes, all six children would have to clean the kitchen because we couldn't agree on whose turn it was. We spent the rest of our Sabbath with each other or visiting the neighbors. Sometimes aunts, uncles, and cousins would drop by for the afternoon. There was no running to the store and dropping by the mall. There were no sports practices or games. It was a day for worship, family, and rest. Not all of my childhood memories are good. Many of them I have had to bury. But my memories of Sundays, our Sabbath Day, are mostly joyous. I often long for the simplicity of those times.

What Happened?

I'm not sure when things changed, but the Sabbath principle is foreign to our modern way of life, even in Bible-belt Christianity. Our mainstream culture is success and profit-driven at all cost. Yes, I do believe that money greed has pushed our society beyond healthy boundaries for good living. Technology has put us on call 24/7. Cell phones, voice mail, email, Facebook, Twitter and all the others have made us way too accessible, in my opinion. It is difficult to resist work, people, and information when it is right in your hand. The virtual world never shuts down and, if you are a progressive person, more than likely you are wired into it. It's probably extremely difficult for you to shut down, too.

I will confess that this is the most difficult commitment for me to keep consistently, mainly because contemporary culture does not acknowledge a need for rest. At best, a weekly day for relaxation and refreshing is tolerated. It is certainly not celebrated. No day is sacred or off limits anymore, as in the past. It is increasingly challenging to say "no" to the lure into some type of activity which keeps us moving at break-neck speed seven days a week.

Because we are violating our body's need for consistent, rhythmic rest, many of us feel just like a toddler who is off her daily routine. We are cranky, irritable, and throw fits. I know I have neglected the Sabbath principle when a simple request, like "pass the salt", makes me burst into tears. It means I have been on "go" for far too many days without 24 hours of reprieve. Armed with the knowledge that I have about my human need for a full day of restoration, I now force myself to stop before I feel this way. I cease my labor. The world can survive without me for one day, including my home, family, and ministry.

Because we are violating our body's need for consistent, rhythmic rest, many of us feel just like a toddler who is off her daily routine.

Although I have not mastered this commitment to keep a weekly Sabbath, just being conscious of it and striving to practice it has helped me manage stress tremendously.

Quick Tips

Here are some tips that may answer some questions you have and help you find and keep *your* Sabbath:

- **Communicate with your household.** If this is something new for you, please communicate with your spouse and/or children that you are working on getting healthier and one of the ways is getting a day of rest each week. This will be really important if they are accustomed to you being the family work-horse who never stops. If you're like me, you created that "super woman" and only you can kill her. Communicating your new commitment with your family is vital. I am sure they love you and will cooperate as best as possible.

- **Define your "rest".** Resting is an individualistic thing and varies from person to person. What refreshes one may drain another. To me, resting is not sleeping all day or lying around watching TV. Both of those actually zap my energy. Rather, it is ceasing from any activity that makes a withdrawal from me. I may do a lot of things on my Sabbath but they are restorative activities that I enjoy and don't call "work". On that day, I purposefully resist meeting demands as an employer, employee, business owner, minister, etc. My mind and spirit get a much needed break.

  "Rest" for me looks like browsing through a boutique, visiting with my family and friends, reading a book, leisurely cooking a meal and working in my flower garden. The point of a day of rest is not ceasing *all* activity, but resisting *work*. What does a day of rest look like to you?

- **Work six days and rest one.** Choose one day out of each week and designate that day as your Sabbath when you will do nothing that you categorize as work. Use this day to relax, refresh, and reflect. Do only those things that are restorative to your mind, body, and soul. As stated earlier, your Sabbath should be unique to you.

> *Your Sabbath should be unique to you.*

Here is a picture of my world and how I use the Sabbath principle. My work is not a typical Monday thru Friday, eight to five job. As a ministry leader, I work often from my home and my hours are not standard, to say the least. Sometimes it seems it would be easier to take a day off if I had a "regular" job. My ministry demands, business work, and household management seem to bleed together and I could easily work all the time. That's one of the detriments of working from home; you're always at work. Then I also live and sleep with my boss and business partner. Then there are the children with needs that never stop. I think you get the picture.

My Sabbath may vary each week; it just depends on the event calendar. Since I have some control over it and I am conscious of my need for a weekly day to rest, I attempt to not over-schedule myself. If I know I have a major weekend event, I will not commit to anything that requires my physical presence or is mentally taxing for the next couple of days. I will use one day to catch up with things in the home and the next day to rest, or vice versa.

You may say, "I don't have that kind of flexibility." Maybe you don't. But what you do have is a God-given right to choose how you will spend your time and live your life. The most self-empowering thing you can do is take ownership of this right. The most self-defeating thing you can do is give this power to something or someone else. Only slaves don't have a choice. If you see clearly your need to rest one day a week, say this aloud right now: I am free to choose how I will live my life. I make the choice to find one day a week to restore my body and mind.

As I said earlier, some weeks I lose my rhythm and a weekly day of rest doesn't happen for me. If I work non-stop for more than seven or eight days in a row, my mood, memory, and creativity suffer tremendously. I imme-

> *If I work non-stop for more than seven or eight days in a row, my mood, memory, and creativity suffer tremendously. I immediately can diagnose the problem—I missed my Sabbath.*

diately can diagnose the problem—I missed my Sabbath.

- **Prepare for the Sabbath.** Here is another tip that I have learned from the Scriptures and put into practice. When God gave the Israelites the command to rest on the seventh day, he instructed them to gather twice as much food on the sixth day so they would have meals for the next. In essence, he told them to prepare for it on the day before. I think this is an important key to keeping the Sabbath: preparation. As I reflect on my growing years in the south, this is exactly what our family did. We hustled on Saturday so we could worship and rest on Sunday.

  Most people I talk to about the Sabbath principle think it's a great idea in theory but don't see how they can take a day to just rest. Women, in particular, are working long hours outside of the home five days a week, which requires them to use their entire weekend to catch up on housework. When I talk to them about a whole day of rest each week they look at me in disbelief; like a deer stuck in the headlights of a car. They just can't see how this is possible. But it is if you make it a priority and *prepare* for it by doing more on your "sixth" day so you can have a day of restoration the next. For example, cook twice as much on the day before your planned Sabbath so the family can eat leftovers the following day; or take the family out to dinner on your rejuvenation day.

Think about the Sabbath like you're going on vacation. You have to work a little bit harder right before you leave town because you know you'll be out of reach for a while. You make sure all the bills are paid; plants are watered, etc., so you don't have to worry about it during your vacation. Well, the Sabbath is your once-a-week, 24 hour holiday. What I know for sure is that if you don't plan it and prepare for it, you won't get it. Planning and preparation are keys to finding and keeping your Sabbath. It's worth it to stay refreshed, pleasant, sharp, and creative.

> *The Sabbath is your once-a-week, 24 hour holiday.*

- **Don't let the Sabbath stress you out.** Please don't think about this as some other thing you've got to put on your "to do" list—#51 Keep the Sabbath. This principle is not intended to stress you but to bless you. It is a Biblical law, but not one to condemn you when you don't keep it. Think of it more as a light that God gave to show us the pathway to great life and productivity: consistent, rhythmic rest for the body. Do the best you can, with the intent to get better at keeping a day of rest each week. Don't stress over it if you miss it. God won't be mad at you. The day benefits you not Him. Just get back on track as soon as possible.

- **Be honest with yourself.** If you cannot find one day a week to stop and be restored, I strongly encourage you to examine what you are doing and why. God created the heavens and the earth in six days and then rested. What are you doing that is so important that you can't rejuvenate one day a week? Why are you doing it? What are you really gaining? Big question . . . what if you died or became very ill? Would things go on without you? Would the world go on without you?

> *If you cannot find one day a week to stop and be restored, I strongly encourage you to examine what you are doing and why.*

Of course, the answer to the final question is yes. The world would move on without all of us. So let it go without you for 24 hours while you take a break. Right now, own your power to choose to rest one day. Don't be a slave to work, money, perfection, performance or achievement any longer. Choose to find and keep your Sabbath—because you can!

I must say this . . .

Many people do see the Sabbath as a Biblical law and not just as a principle. They honor and practice it as a part of their worship to God. I highly respect that and do not intend to lessen the Sabbath by presenting it as optional. The reality is, however, the majority of people in today's society are not conscious of this day at all. My aim is to magnify this powerful commandment God gave us to completely rest one day a week. God's way is always the best way and those who obey have a much greater chance for a longer, stronger and happier life.

> *So there is a special rest still waiting for the people of God. For all who have entered into God's rest have rested from their labors, just as God did after creating the world. So let us do our best to enter that rest. But if we disobey God, as the people of Israel did, we will fall.*
>
> *Hebrews 4:9-11*
> *New Living Translation*

Right Now

Do you recognize a need for a weekly day of restorative rest for your body, mind, and spirit?

What do you need to do differently to make this day possible?

COMMITMENT THREE

I will eat whole foods.

"Let food be thy medicine and medicine be thy food."
Hippocrates

Fighting stress is much greater than easing the mind and resting the spirit. The body must also be fed properly. Researchers are still discovering that nature provides the perfect dietary support for not only a healthy body, but also a strong mind and spirit. Yes, food directly impacts our mental and emotional well-being. When our bodies are properly nourished from nature's bounty, we are able to experience greater joy, fight off sickness, and recover from the harmful effects of stress. Food does so much more than just thrill our senses and fill our bellies. It fuels our life.

Food does so much more than just thrill our senses and fill our bellies. It fuels our life.

In today's fast-paced, profit-driven, "get-it-to-market quickly" world, much of what we call food has been so processed that it is not really food at all. It may fill our stomachs and satisfy our hunger, but it provides very little nourishment for our body. If your diet consists mostly of manufactured, over-processed food, your body is not equipped with what it needs to recover from stress. Junk food, as we call it, is just that—cheap and worthless when it comes to supplying the body with the necessary energy to thrive.

Whole vs. Organic

Whole foods are unprocessed or unrefined—or minimally processed. They do not contain manufactured ingredients such as preservatives, antibiotics, dyes, and other chemicals. Whole foods are sometimes called all-natural. Organic foods and whole foods are different. Organic means they are grown without synthetic pesticides and other chemical assistance. All-natural foods are not necessarily organic. For example, an apple is definitely a whole food, but not all apples are organically grown.

The absolute best things you can eat are those which are grown without pesticides and other chemicals, but as a start you should focus on getting more all-natural foods in your diet. Don't over-pressure yourself to eat organically, especially if you have been living a junk-food lifestyle for a long time. Just begin with eating less processed things out of packages and getting more whole foods into your body. You will be amazed at how a healthier daily menu can help fight the effects of stress and lengthen your life.

A Yam Saved My Life

Nature heals us. I received this revelation a few years ago after the birth of our sixth daughter. I became very ill a few days after she was born. I began to have extreme anxiety, panic, sleeplessness, recurring infections and fainting spells. My obstetrician didn't know what was wrong with me and we felt pretty hopeless for an answer. One evening, in a fit of desperation, my husband called the home of a doctor in Kansas City, who we only knew from a distance at the time. Thank God, she took the call at home and asked me a series of questions about my symptoms. She made several other queries, of which I didn't understand the relevance but answered anyway.

"How old are you, Genette? How many children do you have? What are their ages? How many years are between each of them?"

I answered each question: I was 37 years old and had six children, ages 11, 9, 6, two "almost" 3, and a newborn—all girls. I had delivered six kids in an eleven year span. The children before my newborn are identical twins. I candidly told her what I was experiencing, even the parts I was ashamed of—like not being able to tolerate the sound of the twins crying and being afraid that I would harm them. I was in a very dark place that I had never known. Thank God I had people to help me care for the children and did not have to manage them alone.

She listened intently and emerged with a very confident response. She said that more than likely I was suffering from a depletion of progesterone. Honestly, I don't think I had even heard of progesterone at that point so I certainly didn't know what it was or how it impacted my life. She slowly explained to me that progesterone is a hormone which is produced in the placenta and is vital in the reproductive process. After the birth of a baby, the body's progesterone passes with the placenta. Typically, the hormone's levels are replenished over time after pregnancy. Because I had birthed so many babies in a short period of time, it could have been possible that my progesterone never restored to adequacy. Then she explained the power of hormones in general and the impact they have on almost every bodily function, including appetite, mood, sleep patterns, and the ability to fight disease. She felt certain that things would turn around for me with hormonal supplementation and proper nutrition.

I will never forget my conversation with her as she went over my treatment plan. She said, "Genette, I am going to send you the hormone supplementation you need that is bio-identical to progesterone. It is found in a yam."

"Huh?" I said. "Yam . . . as in sweet potato?"

She chuckled. "Yes. Yam, as in a sweet potato."

I was stunned. Who knew that a yam had hormones in it? She also instructed me to take a whole food vitamin and mineral supplement every morning and to try to eat as organically as possible. She emphasized how critical it was to watch my nutrition. I was desperate to get well for the sake of my husband and children so I followed her instructions to the letter. With my husband as my coach and overseer, I daily took my sublingual hormonal therapy (from a yam!), whole food supplements, and ate only the foods that God created, in their most unrefined form. In a matter of weeks, I was thriving.

The healing miracle I needed was in a yam. It was also in the host of fruits, vegetables, grains, and other organically-grown foods I ate. That still amazes me. That health crisis taught me the power of nature and started me on the path to life-long wellness. Now food is my medicine and I am conscious of everything that I put in my body.

The truth is this: our bodies are just like any other equipment. In order for it to function properly, we must give it the fuel it needs. God has given us everything we need in this earth to survive and thrive. When we feed our bodies the proper nutrition, we are able to heal, fight off sickness and also the harmful effects of stress.

When we feed our bodies the proper nutrition, we are able to heal, fight off sickness and also the harmful effects of stress.

The Food and Stress Dilemma

The dilemma with food and stress is that when we are we under duress we often crave junk food. This is probably because stress drains the body's energy stores.

With our fast-paced lifestyles, we tend to reach for quick fixes to our low energy levels, such as caffeine and sweets. We may get a short-lived energy burst but we quickly crash and burn. The junk food actually makes us more sluggish, uncomfortable, and irritable than we were before. It's a vicious cycle that must be broken with knowledge and discipline.

Seven Nutrition Essentials for Fighting Stress

I am not a physician or nutritionist, but I am a committed life-long learner about nutrition and wellness now. From my research, there are seven nutrition essentials that our bodies need to help reduce the effects of stress. These are found in abundance in nature, but in very few cans, boxes, or other packaging. Eating fresh, whole foods is the key to getting these nutrients. You should also note that none of these nutrients is manufactured in the body. They must be supplied in our diet or through supplementation.

> *None of these nutrients is manufactured in the body. They must be supplied in our diet or through supplementation.*

Vitamins C & E—Fight free radical damage caused by stress

When you are stressed your body releases more free radicals than usual. Free radicals are atoms with an unpaired number of molecules. They enter the body seeking to attach themselves to your DNA and cause damage, called oxidation. Excessive free radical damage can severely break down the body's immune system. This is why you have a tendency to get sick when you are under extreme stress.

Vitamins C and E are the most powerful anti-oxidation nutrients that combat free radical damage.

Here are foods that are loaded with Vitamins C and E:

Vitamin C—the citrus family (oranges, grapefruit, lemons and limes), green peppers, cabbage, spinach, broccoli, kale, cantaloupe, kiwi, and strawberries.

Vitamin E—nuts, seeds, vegetable and fish oils, whole grains (especially wheat germ), and apricots.

Vitamin B Family—Weaves a web for overall well-being

There are eleven members of the vitamin B family and together they are known as B-complex. They are critical nutrients to every mind-related function, especially mood and memory function. They also assist with the production of energy for the body. The B-complex family is involved behind the scenes in an intricate way in the production of serotonin, metabolism of fat and even the repair of damaged DNA. It is essential that you have proper intake of B-complex daily, but especially when you are under a season of unusual stress.

Here are foods you should eat to supply B vitamins in your diet:

Protein from animal sources such as fish, beef, and poultry; dark green vegetables and whole grains

Magnesium—Relaxes the muscles

Magnesium is known as the anti-stress nutrient because it relaxes the body's muscles, including the heart and bowel muscles. Magnesium can slow down heart palpitations brought on by stress. It also helps with eliminating toxins from the body because it relaxes the bowels. It has a calming effect on the entire body and helps with deeper sleep. Magnesium in proper dosages fights against depression, anxiety, panic attacks, insomnia, high blood pressure, and abnormal heart beats. All of these are in some way stress-induced.

These are the power foods that are rich in magnesium:

Seafood, dark greens, beans, grains, nuts and seeds

L-Tryptophan—Triggers the "feel-good" hormones

L-Tryptophan is an essential amino acid that causes the release of serotonin and melatonin into the body. These are two of the "feel-good" hormones, or neurotransmitters, in the brain. They are commonly known to attribute to our ability to feel happy. They also contribute to our sleep and overall sense of well-being.

Protein and dairy are typically foods rich in L-Tryptophan:

Turkey, chicken, seafood, cheese, yogurt, beans, and cashews

Protein—Stabilizes blood sugar and mood swings

Fluctuating blood sugar levels are not only detrimental to the waist-line, but also to the mood. A sudden swing in blood sugar levels can cause irritability, anger, depression, and stress. Protein greatly helps with stabilizing blood sugar levels, minimizing food-induced mood swings. A diet that is rich in lean proteins not only produces a stronger and leaner body, but a better mental disposition.

Protein rich foods are not only meats, but also:

Eggs, cheese, dairy, beans, nuts, grains, and tofu

Fiber—Sweeps wastes and toxins out of the body

Toxins are a part of our everyday existence. When they linger too long in the body, they slow us down. They also hamper the body's ability to heal and fight disease, including stress. Fiber is essential because it provides the digestive tract with the force it needs to flush away toxins. When we are not properly getting rid of waste, we become sluggish, lethargic, and irritable. Fiber also helps stabilize blood sugar.

Here are some fiber-rich foods you should include in your diet:

Fruits (especially apples, oranges, pears, and berries), colorful vegetables, whole grains (especially oats), nuts, and seeds

Water—Hydrates the body

Proper hydration is critical to every function in the body. It is essential to life. Even a mild case of dehydration can stress the entire body. Paradoxically, stress itself dehydrates the body. Dehydration affects thinking, causes nausea, and headaches. The worse-case scenario of sustained dehydration is death. When you are under extreme stress, it is critical that you drink plenty of pure water. Take in the life.

Quick Tips

I'm a busy mother of six and eating healthy meals with lean protein, fruits, and vegetables is a daily challenge. Some days I don't hit the target, but most days I do. Here are some simple things I practice, along with a few of my go-to foods, that may help you in your quest to eat healthier:

1. **Become a life-long label reader.** It is critical that you know what you are putting in your body, especially if it comes in a package. So before you put it in your mouth, read the label for the ingredients. If you cannot pronounce most of them, I highly recommend you don't eat it. They are probably some form of preservative, dye, food substitute, or artificial flavor enhancer. The FDA allows these chemicals in food because they are not harmful in miniscule amounts. However, if consumed consistently and over a length of time, these substances compound in the body and can cause all kinds of problems. If it's in a package, please read it before you eat it.

2. **Become a life-long learner.** Ignorance is not bliss when it comes to nutrition. Discoveries are still being made concerning beneficial foods and harmful additives. Subscribe to nutrition and wellness periodicals to stay aware of the latest findings. I find that being knowledgeable empowers me to make better choices in my food selection. When I read the labels, I cannot only identify the harmful substances but I also know the potential effect they have on my body. Knowledge is power, but applying the knowledge is wisdom. Be wise.

3. **Keep a whole food supplement in sight.** A whole food supplement is a combination of vitamins and minerals that are extracted from raw fruits and vegetables. If you talk to 100 nutrition experts you will probably get 100

different recommendations on the supplements you "must" take daily. The one that will probably be on every list is a whole food multivitamin/ mineral. This is where I suggest you start if you are a beginner in the wellness lifestyle. Don't put them in the cabinet—out of sight, out of mind. Put them within your eyesight and easy reach each day. You may even consider starting out with a gummie or chewable whole food supplement, especially if you have difficulty swallowing pills. Just pop it in your mouth and chew as you walk out of the door.

4. **Follow the 80-20 rule.** Yes, the Pareto principle even holds true for nutrition, according to research. The Pareto law states that 80% of the effects come from 20% of the causes. Nutritionally this means that 20% of your diet is probably causing 80% of your problems. If you are struggling with your weight, for example, it is probably because 20% of the foods you are eating are loaded with fat, sugar, and calories of no nutritional content. If you can identify and eliminate these foods, your weight will begin to drop dramatically. Remember, it's roughly only 20% of your diet. So you don't have to change everything. Just the problem foods. On the other hand, if you can identify several nutritionally dense foods you enjoy (lean proteins, fruit, vegetables, and grains) and eat these 80% of the time, you will be on your way to great health. The other 20% of the time, splurge on some junk you may be craving.

For example, my 20% vice is sugar and baked goods. They cause me 80% of my weight control problems. I apply the 80-20 rule by restricting them during the weekdays, and sticking to a diet of my favorite lean proteins, fruits, veggies, nuts, etc. On the weekends, I allow myself a sweet treat or whatever I want.

5. **Eat your calories. Don't drink them.** If you are a heavy soda, juice, and sweet tea drinker, you are consuming a significant number of empty calories that are expanding your waistline, slowing you down, and impairing your body's ability to fight stress. The average sweetened beverage has 150 calories per serving. If you have one soda with each meal, that's a whopping 450 calories per day on drinking, not eating. As for me, I'd much rather eat that 450 calories and pair it with a glass of zero calorie, refreshing water, that my body desperately needs. Make water your beverage of choice with each meal and you should see a significant decrease in your waistline, increase in your energy, and stabilization of your mood.

6. **Here are a few of my go-to foods that are quick, easy and nutritionally sound for stress-relief:**

    • A handful of nuts. The best are almonds.

    • Apples, oranges, grapefruit, and berries of all types. Eat bananas in moderation because they are heavy in sugar.

- All natural peanut butter on whole grain bread

- Mixed salad with protein on top

- Boiled eggs

- All natural cheeses

- Popcorn (my FAVORITE snack)

- Tortilla chips and salsa or guacamole

My fast food favorites:

- Oatmeal with fruit from McDonald's and Starbucks

- "Power" breakfast sandwiches from Panera Bread and Starbucks

- Salads with grilled chicken from McDonald's, Wendy's, and Chick-fil-a

- Subway turkey sandwich on whole wheat

I Must Say This . . .

God has given us everything we need in abundance to live long and strong lives. It is found in the huge variety and supply of foods in the earth. The flavor combinations are endline. Eating is meant to be a pleasurable experience, so taste matters. Enjoy yourself and eat until you are content. Just eat *food*—things that grow from nature—not science projects that come down manufacturing lines. You will be amazed at how

Enjoy yourself and eat until you are content. Just eat food—things that grow from nature—not science projects that come down manufacturing lines.

good real food tastes and you won't want to go back to the junk food life. Eat to your good health.

Right Now

Can you identify foods in your diet that may be short-circuiting your body's ability to fight the deadly effects of stress?

What are your favorite vegetables, fruits, and protein or lean meats? Can you commit to increase these—little by little—in your diet?

Do you take a whole food supplement daily or consistently? If not, when will you begin?

COMMITMENT FOUR

I will move my body.

"I now know my body was made to move, not park. The more I move it, the better I feel. Energy creates energy."
—*Genette Howard*

The first argument I had with my husband, Dexter, was in a gym. We were engaged to be married and took our first trip together to the fitness club. He was training for NFL tryouts and I was trying to lose a few pounds so I could look svelte in my borrowed wedding gown. I was 125 pounds and a perfect size six. Unfortunately, my girlfriend's gown was a four. The seamstress let it out as far as it could go and I needed to lose a couple of inches in the midsection to be more comfortable. That was before Spanx and the other miracle garments we have now. Had they been available back then, I certainly would have taken that option and saved myself from the ugly episode I had with my sweet fiancé. But I guess I had to learn.

Dexter and I were a match made in heaven and shared most things in common—except a love of exercise and sweat. I was a certified PYT (pretty young thing) who never participated in a sport. I had never pushed my body to the brink because there was no need to. I ate what I wanted and maintained a small physique. I was not motivated to torture myself with running, jumping, kicking, and lifting until I could barely breathe. I had tried working out a few times with college friends because they seemed to enjoy it but I never lasted. Truthfully, I hated exercising. I would rather shop, read, decorate, cook, clean . . . anything . . . than exercise.

This is the girl who walked into the gym with her NFL-training fiancé. The whining began after the first warm-up lap and got worse each minute. His gentle motivating eventually turned into frustration, then anger as I complained, resisted, and finally refused to do one more lift, squat, rep, or stretch. I was tired and I wasn't moving another muscle. The more he explained that my legs were *supposed* to be shaking, my arms were *supposed* to burn, and my heart was *supposed* to feel like it was going to beat out of my chest, the angrier I got. I thought he was trying to kill me. He thought I was pretty pitiful. It turned ugly and we both drove home in silence. That was 18 years ago and not much has changed with me when it comes to pushing my body to its limit.

As a matter of fact, the word "exercise" is an immediate turn off to me. It conjures up an image of a stinky gym with big, intimidating equipment I don't know how to use. Or, my mind turns toward pain. I don't like pain. If you invite me to "exercise" with you, you will most likely get an excuse of why I can't come. Oddly enough, I have managed to maintain a healthy weight and strong body, even after birthing six children. While I am not an avid exerciser, I am a woman who moves her body, consistently and intentionally. I finally made the connection that what is commonly known as "exercising" or "working out" is just vigorous movement of the body over a sustained period of time. I dropped the dread and picked up activities

> *What is commonly known as "exercising" or "working out" is just vigorous movement of the body over a sustained period of time.*

I love. It has made all the difference in maintaining an active lifestyle. If you don't love it, you'll probably leave it. So do what you love.

Love It or Leave It

My body movement of choice is dancing. I have always loved moving to music. I can hardly resist a pulsating rhythm. Something in me just has to move. So I am an enthusiastic Jazzercizer. It's serious cardio, strength training and stretching to popular music for one hour. But my mind does not register it as dreaded exercise. I'm having fun as I work my large and small muscle groups to the pumping beats. With sweat dripping down my back, I sing the lyrics when I can catch my breath. I leave all the cares of my world behind for an hour as I focus on the music and the movements. On the routines I have down pat, I get a little jiggy with it just because I can. Here I have found my love of music, dancing, and inspiration. I look forward to every session.

I also enjoy walking in the spring when the flowers are first blooming, and in the fall, when the trees are showing off their foliage. Beauty ministers deeply to my soul, so I speed-walk through my manicured, hilly neighborhood and take it all in. I'm not even conscious of the mist on my brow and my flexing hamstrings as I'm communing with my Father and His creation. I'm just engaging with things I love—nature, beautiful homes, and God's goodness.

For my birthday a couple of years ago, my church congregation bought me a bike from a high-end shop. I refuse to let it sit in my garage because it was costly. So I ride it on care-free days and I feel like a kid again. My husband requested one for his birthday and now we ride together on the trails every chance we get. I don't know how many calories I burn, but the light-hearted moments and memories we create on those bikes are priceless. Our favorite cycling adventure together was when the overcast summer sky turned into a much-needed rain shower as we rode along a trail. We began to pedal fast like 12 year olds trying to get home before dark. We were tired, wet, cool, and happy when we finally found where we parked the car. Our bike rides are much more than physical conditioning. They are refreshing to our mind, spirit, and relationship.

I know they say, "no pain, no gain." I understand that when it comes to building muscle and re-shaping the body. But as it relates to stress-relief, I believe discovering physical activity you actually enjoy is what is most important—if for no other reason than you will look forward to it and stick with it. It's what we do most consistently that has the most impact. When you see something as drudgery or associate it with pain, it is highly de-motivating. More than likely, the pain will overpower you, excuses will set in, and you'll fizzle out. It's human nature to run from pain and toward pleasure. Find what you love.

I live a joyful life and I believe it is because I have freed myself to do what I'm passionate about. I resist the pressure to conform to anything I really don't enjoy—especially if I have a choice. I know that my best results will come from sticking with my unique, divine design and preferences.

Body Movement and Stress Relief

I believe this is what really counts when it comes to stress relief—movement of the body and engagement of the muscles for sustained periods of time in *any kind* of activity that you enjoy. An active lifestyle is vital to overall health, happiness, and a sense of well-being. The body is like a machine and it was created to move. We know the weight-reduction benefits of actively moving the body, but body movement is also significantly helpful in combating the affects of stress.

> *We know the weight-reduction benefits of actively moving the body, but body movement is also significantly helpful in combating the affects of stress.*

Here are some of the most significant stress-reducing results of physical exercise. Remember, physical exercise is *any kind* of movement of the body for a sustained period of time.

- **Release of endorphins.** Endorphins are among the "feel good" hormones released by the brain. Your body's production of endorphins increase during vigorous physical activity. Endorphins give you a sense of well-being and brighten your outlook.

- **Mental relaxation**. I heard someone say that when the body is in movement, the mind is at rest. When you focus in on some sort of vigorous activity, your mind is distracted from worry, anxious thoughts, and negative feelings. The mind gets a much needed break.

- **Sense of accomplishment.** Anytime we complete a task, meet a goal, or overcome a challenge, we feel strong and empowered. Conversely, inactivity breeds more inactivity, which makes us feel lousy about ourselves and our situation. Intentionally moving the body—if just dancing around in the floor—can break the cycle of lethargy and feelings of hopelessness.

- **Better health.** Of course the benefits of body movement to our overall health are endless. Exercise is vital to losing weight and maintaining a healthy weight; building and maintaining a healthy heart; keeping muscles and bones healthy;

relieving pain; improving sleep; and increasing immunity to sicknesses. These are just a few of the health benefits of physical activity. When our overall health increases we are a lot less subject to sickness. Sickness and disease are major life stressors. A strong body helps keep you well and checks this type of stress at the door.

> *When our overall health increases we are a lot less subject to sickness. Sickness and disease are major life stressors.*

Stretching and Stress Reduction

Stretching is a form of exercise and has powerful stress-relieving benefits. Some of the most popular stretching regimens are Yoga and Pilates. Yoga, Pilates, and other regimens combine stretching with deep breathing because they work in tandem for best results, particularly for stress relief. Any fitness expert would highly recommend these because of their undeniable benefits to the body. However you don't have to take a Yoga or Pilates class to stretch your muscles. Just a few simple moves each day, with deep breathing, can help release stress from the body and give instant relief.

Stress tends to gather in the neck, shoulders, and back causing tight, sore muscles. Overtime the unreleased stress develops into toxic "knots". Here are the ways that stretching helps to rid the body of these deadly knots:

- **Stretching increases blood circulation.** The blood carries the life of the body. Stretching specific areas of the body send the flow of blood where it is needed most. Blood circulation is vital to stress relief.

- **Stretching induces deeper breathing, which sends more oxygen through the body.** This helps with slowing the heart rate and increases the mind's ability to relax.

- **Stretching loosens the muscles.** Loose muscles help in the release of toxic knots.

- **Stretching suppresses the production of harmful stress hormones,** like cortisol, while increasing the production of the anti-depressant hormones like dopamine, serotonin, and norepinephrine.

Quick Tips

I am committed to an active lifestyle because I believe it honors God when we use the body He has given us to actively engage in life. This is the mindset I have adopted and it helps to stay physically active. Here are some of the simple things I intentionally do to keep my body moving:

It honors God when we use the body He has given us to actively engage in life.

1. Dancing—anytime for any reason

2. Short and long power walks

3. 200 jumping jacks in the morning and/or evening

4. Side bends, leg, arm and neck stretches in the morning and/or evening

5. Push-ups and sit-ups in the morning and/or evening

6. Stair climbing in my home and at work

7. Bike rides

8. Long shopping excursions at the mall(s)

9. Yard work

10. Housework for one hour

11. Escapades with my husband (yes, sex!)

Now think about your daily lifestyle and activities:

Do you have stairs in your home? Intentionally go up and down them several times until your heart rate increases. Maybe you can do this while you're also doing housework, like putting away laundry. Make several trips on purpose. Run the stairs if you can.

Do you have stairs at your workplace? Intentionally find reasons to go up and down those stairs each day.

The key is to get your heart rate up and begin breathing more deeply.

Do you live in a neighborhood with great walking trails or hills? Take advantage of it. A brisk 15 to 20 minute walk on a hilly trail is plenty to get your heart going and release the endorphins.

Do you love to shop? You will be surprised at how many steps you take during a day-long shopping excursion. Use the "shop 'til you drop" principle to your physical advantage. Keep it moving from store to store.

Do you have a lawn or garden to maintain? Yard work is great exercise. Beautify your home while you move your body and fight stress.

Do you have little kids? Feed off of their boundless energy and play with them. Turn on some silly music and dance in the middle of the floor for a few songs. They will love you even more and you will get the endorphin rush you need to fight stress.

Do you have a spouse? When you are under duress, it is not abnormal for your libido to decrease because chronic stress wreaks havoc on hormonal levels. It may take a little bit more to get you warmed up, but I encourage you to do whatever it takes to stay in the swing of things sexually. Sex is a great exercise and the nurturing afterwards greatly helps women in particular with stress-relief.

Do you love to dance? I believe it is impossible to dance and be sad at the same time. Dancing is for joy! I take advantage of every opportunity I get to dance—with my husband, kids, and friends. I encourage you to do the same. With or without a partner, crank up your favorite music and dance, dance, dance! Create your own atmosphere of happiness, joy and celebration because you are alive.

I must say this . . .

Out of all my years of resisting exercise and work outs, I am grateful that I have finally picked up an active lifestyle that includes sweating and stretching. I enjoy looking good, but for me the best result of consistent physical activity is not a smaller waistline, but a greater sense of well-being. I once had to have frequent massages and chiropractic therapy on my neck and shoulders because the tension knots were so severe. At one point, I did not have full mobility of my neck. Now I feel no need for chiropractic care and have massages for pleasure and maintenance—not because I can barely move my neck or shoulders. I now know my body was made to move, not park. The more I move it, the better I feel. Energy creates energy.

> *I now know my body was made to move, not park. The more I move it, the better I feel. Energy creates energy.*

"Training the body helps a little, but godly living helps in every way. Godly living has the promise of life now and in the world to come."

I Timothy 4:8
God's Word Translation

Right Now

What physical activities do you enjoy? Do you sweat when you do them?

Do you have a regular stretching routine?

From the suggestions I gave, what simple things can you do to get your heart pumping at least 3 times per week for 20 to 30 minutes?

COMMITMENT FIVE

I will spend time with my friends.

"A friend is a present you give yourself."
Robert Louis Stevenson

On June 4, 1994, I took my wedding vows at 24 years old and immersed myself wholeheartedly into being a helpmate to my husband. I was smitten by his deep faith in God and powerful calling. I felt honored to be the special lady in his life and willingly surrendered my personal goals and dreams to help him fulfill his. Then the babies began to come—one girl after another—until our quiver was full with six of them. When I finally came up for air 15 years later, I liked what I saw around me—a faithful husband, happy kids, beautiful home and good reputation. But when I looked within me, there was a deep sense of unhappiness.

As I approached 40, it seemed that all of my unfulfilled desires began slapping me in the face and wouldn't stop. I couldn't ignore them any longer. I had to look deep within and confront my discontentment with my life. I was in a major life transition (some call it mid-life crisis) and it was frightening, not only to me, but also to my husband. He could see that I had taken my personal happiness off the backburner and moved it up to the front. As he says, "the heat got hot" as I began to re-discover my passions, desires, and dreams. Had I not been deeply rooted in my faith and God's Word, my self-discovery would have easily turned into selfishness and caused great harm to my family. I know many women who have done things they eventually regretted as they walked through this common transition in life.

My Sad Years

I was suffering from 15 years of self-inflicted neglect. Literally, I just forgot about myself. There it is—the answer to my most frequently asked question: how do you do it? When resources were short—money, time, energy—I used it all to meet the needs of my husband, children, and ministry. Somebody had to sacrifice and I volunteered myself. It was a learned behavior. This is what I saw my mother do so it was the only way I knew to respond to the overwhelming demands of my life. I watched my mom go to work in the factory; come home to cook and clean; meet most of the needs of six kids; worry about bills . . . on and on . . . most of her life. Sadly, I have very few memories of her enjoying herself. To this day she is still suffering from self-neglect.

I call those 15 years "my sad years" because now I know that most of the things I sacrificed were not only unnecessary, but unwise. The one that I regret the most is losing contact with great friends. You see, I am not a loner. Before I took on the "wife/mom/minister" roles, I was rolling with my girls. My first girlfriend was my big sister, Angela. Even though she was three years older, we were like two peas in the pod and did everything together. Our family life was volatile so we were comfort for each other. We were exposed to too much trouble early in life so we would spend hours talking like two

Now I know that most of the things I sacrificed were not only unnecessary, but unwise.

old women about men, bills, and "these bad kids" while we combed our doll's hair, sewed our hand-made purses, and made mud pies. When she left for college I cried for days as I had to adjust to sleeping in a bed without her.

As I grew up, I had close friends from all walks of life who I deeply enjoyed. My list of girlfriends I could call to go shopping, grab a bite to eat, or just shoot the breeze was long. I loved having friends and being a friend. It was a simple source of pleasure that I felt I couldn't afford anymore as my responsibilities grew.

Now I am intentionally re-connecting with dear friends who are scattered all over the world. I remember the remorse I felt when one of them confessed that she had felt slighted by me. She thought I had dropped her friendship because I had become too important. She eventually stopped reaching out to me. I had to hold back tears as I walked her through my sad years of survival and self-neglect. Then I affirmed to her my love, admiration, and desperate need for friendship.

The Science of Intimacy and Stress-Relief

New scientific research revealed to me that the deep sense of unhappiness that surfaced around 40 was partly related to my void of intimate friendship with other women. My years of loneliness were also working against my body's ability to fight stress. For women, in particular, spending intimate time with friends is not a luxury but a necessity for healthy living.

> *For women, in particular, spending intimate time with friends is not a luxury but a necessity for healthy living.*

During my mid-life transition, I picked up a book called "Venus on Fire, Mars on Ice" by famed relationship expert and author Dr. John Gray. You probably have read or heard of his best-selling book "Men are From Mars, Women are From Venus". I was drawn by the cover art which was an animated illustration of a man and woman sitting as far apart as possible on the sofa with their backs turned on each other. He is wearing a heavy coat, hat and earmuffs and she is wearing a sundress, shades, and flip flops. He's cold and she's sweating while fanning away a hot flash. They obviously are unhappy with each other, avoiding touching at all costs. I chuckled because it was a pretty accurate depiction of my marriage at the time. I purchased it in hopes it would shed some light on the challenging transition my life and relationship was in—and it did.

Dr. Gray shares groundbreaking research that reveals that men and women are different, not just in our communication styles, but all the way down to the cellular level. Our biochemistry is worlds apart. He shows that much of the major conflict between today's man and woman is due to unparalleled stress, which has thrown the delicate hormonal balance in both sexes severely out-of-whack. Men and women are in a fight to survive, and ironically, the biochemistry

> *Much of the major conflict between today's man and woman is due to unparalleled stress, which has thrown the delicate hormonal balance in both sexes severely out-of-whack.*

of stress-reduction for them is worlds apart. Literally, the activities that help the sexes fight stress are polar opposites and can create major conflict when they are not understood.

Here is a quick synopsis of the differences in male and female biochemistry as it relates to stress. As you may know, testosterone is the major hormone in men, and its primary function is to increase sex drive and aggression. But that's not the whole truth about testosterone. It is also the hormone in men that helps them relax and fight stress. When a man has worked a full day of physical or mental labor, his testosterone levels have been depleted. The primary way a man's testosterone levels are restored is through rest. Yes, Lazy Boy, remote control, cave-time rest. The recliner is really not as much about laziness as it is about survival for a man. Instinctively, he is drawn to rest after hard work because his body needs to restore testosterone levels to fight stress and survive. The key to remember is that testosterone is the man's stress-fighting hormone and it is replenished by rest.

The stress-fighting hormone in women is oxytocin. Oxytocin is released and replenished when a woman engages in any kind of nurturing activities. A very common activity that releases oxytocin is nursing a baby. I nursed all six of our children and I recall falling asleep almost immediately at each feeding session. That's the power of oxytocin. It is THE relaxation hormone for women and we instinctively gravitate toward nurturing activities because of our body's need for oxytocin to fight stress. At the end of a long day of physical or mental labor, a woman instinctively searches to unwind by sharing feelings about the day. It is not just an emotional need for women; it is a physiological need.

In today's marriages where both parties are working outside the home and highly stressed, men and women are in survival mode. He needs *rest* to rebuild his stress-fighting testosterone and she needs to *relate* to replenish her stress-fighting oxytocin. The last thing he wants to do when he is feeling stressed is to talk.

> *He needs rest to rebuild his stress-fighting testosterone and she needs to relate to replenish her stress-fighting oxytocin.*

His biochemistry requires him to find the closest cave and shut it all down. Yet, her biochemistry requires some kind of nurturing activity to get her oxytocin flowing. She wants to talk . . . or listen . . . or touch and be touched. If you're married, I imagine this has created some level of conflict in your marriage. Neither one of you is wrong.

You both are trying to get your survival needs met. Unfortunately, they are very different.

Here is a quick solution that works well in my marriage now that we both have this understanding of what the other needs. I give my husband his undisturbed rest time (we call it "cave time") when he gets home in the evening. It's usually about an hour or so. After we finish the evening meal and get the kids settled, we meet on the sofa and I get to have cuddle and relating time. Sometimes we talk. Most times I lay in his lap or on his shoulder as we both stare brainlessly at the TV and comment here or there. Just the closeness is enough to get my oxytocin-fix from him. It works like magic and we both get our needs met.

When Men Aren't Enough

After 18 years of marriage, this is what I know for sure: even the most sensitive man has a threshold when it comes to conversation and verbally relating with other human beings. They simply are not wired to handle the volume of things most women need or want to talk about. That's why I believe every woman needs at least one girlfriend—to hold the spillage of conversation that her man just can't

> *Even the most sensitive man has a threshold when it comes to conversation and verbally relating with other human beings. They simply are not wired to handle the volume of things most women need or want to talk about.*

hold. A girlfriend can handle the details. We specialize in talking about the little things. The borders of our conversations are much greater than men's. A girlfriend has the capacity to hold all of the great "nothings" you need to talk about—like eyebrow waxing, nail polish colors, platform shoes, or your latest favorite thing. Nothing's too big or small. She is there to catch the extras that just won't fit in your man's packaging.

Back in the "good old days", it was a common occurrence for the women to get together in the kitchen to prepare a meal. They would talk—mostly gossip—and laugh up a storm while frying chicken, mixing cakes, rolling out dough . . . what great memories. Oftentimes they would make the little girls leave the kitchen if the conversation would get too hot. My older sister, Angela, was always the one that would get in trouble for hiding out in a corner so she wouldn't miss anything. Those women were socially suppressed but you couldn't tell it by the joy and laughter that was in the kitchen. They were having a great time as they related to each other and prepared a delicious meal to nurture their men and children. They were talking, laughing and cooking to their good health—their oxytocin levels rising off the charts to help them fight their stress.

This scenario is true even in tribal communities, where the roles are more instinctively assigned. While the men relax around the fire, the women talk and laugh with each other as they busily prepare the evening meal. Both sexes are doing what they are physiologically programmed to do to survive. The men are resting to fight the stresses of the day. The women are relating and nurturing to fight theirs. It boils down to testosterone and oxytocin—the stress fighting hormones in men and women.

My Special Gift

The first way I confronted the unhappiness I faced a few years ago was in prayer. I poured out my desires and needs to my Father and he is still answering my prayers for fulfillment in my life. One year ago I received a very special gift from him in the form of my best friend coming back to town. It was such a profound experience for me that I wrote a blog about it that many have enjoyed. I think it is appropriate to share here:

Every Woman Needs a BFF:
Beautiful. Faithful. Friend.

I'm a little hesitant to write this blog because it's deeply personal for me. I'm a pretty transparent person and don't mind sharing my personal experiences if they will help someone. But this one makes me feel a little vulnerable, for some reason. Before I do anything, I generally consider the feelings of others. So my vulnerability may be that I don't want to alienate anyone as I expose my deep appreciation for my BFF—beautiful, faithful, friend. I won't call her name, but if you're from around these parts, it won't take you long to figure it out.

She moved back to town a couple of months ago with a grand entrance and public celebration. Nine years ago, she moved away with her family when her famed hubby got a new job. I was glad for their promotion, but I was heartbroken for myself. Her friendship was like a warm blanket for me. I cannot find the words to articulate the dimensions of our fellowship. It was complete love, acceptance, support, and celebration of each other. When she moved away, it left a void that I never attempted to fill with any other friend. Maybe I thought it was impossible so I never tried. I busied myself with my husband, children, family, and ministry. Besides, the need for a BFF at my age is really petty, I tried to convince myself.

Of course, we still kept in contact over the years with conversations that were not frequent but EXTREMELY long. My husband would sometimes come in the room with a look of disbelief that I was STILL on the phone with the same person. There was just too much to catch up on . . . new nail polish colors, fashion trends, husband issues, kids, money, world crises, Jesus Christ. No topic was too big or too small. Our conversations were borderless.

When I got the call that after nine years they were headed back to town for her husband to take his dream job, I was overjoyed for them! It was a dream—actually, a prophecy—come true. The whole state was in celebration that they were coming home for her husband to lead our beloved team to glory. To watch it all happen with the inside perspective over the years, was such a lesson in the faithfulness of God.

*What surprised me is that so many people were congratulating **me**. They were happy for **me**. I didn't understand that part. Now I do. They saw what I didn't* *see. Or maybe I wouldn't allow myself to see it. My beloved friend was coming home to me. She was back. My ace. My confidante. My BFF. My warm blanket. It was my gift from God and right on time for this season of my life. Now I get it and this is what I want to share with you.*

True friendship is a gift—a priceless gift from God. "A true friend sticks closer than family," Proverbs says. Family is bound by blood but a true friend is bound only by love.

This is the gift I have received and am thoroughly enjoying since she has returned. The simultaneous depth and triviality of our times together are treasures in my heart. It has restored my soul in ways I am still discovering. The lesson I'm learning: you never outgrow the need for a BFF. They are a joy . . . at any age and phase of life.

I don't know if men feel this way about friends. To me it sounds a little too mushy for their metal. I asked my hubby if men had "BFFs" and he replied, "If we do we don't call them that." Just as I thought. Of course, men value friendship, but for women I think the valuation is different. Our well-being seems to be rooted in the quality of our relationships. Husbands are the ultimate prize for a woman, but our girl friends are so vital because they hold the spill-over of all the conversations and feelings our husbands can't hold. They have their limits. That's why every woman needs a beautiful, faithful friend.

Friendship is not possession. I have many friends who I love and so does my BFF. I'm open to new friends and welcome them. But new friendships take time and effort to develop. Sometimes it's worth it. Sometimes it's not. The gift of a BFF is that the waters have already been tested. Your soul can rest with them. You can be as small or great as you want to be around them. They can handle all of you. They welcome all of you. What a gift.

I pray for you today that your soul would find a resting place like this with a friend. I pray that you grow in your capacity to give and receive this kind of friendship—unselfish, untwisted, unperverted, faithful, and loyal. In Jesus' precious name. Amen.

Quick Tips

Today's women are busier than ever before in history, moving at break-neck speeds to meet the demands of work, home, and other arenas. It's easy to begin sacrificing the simple pleasures of life, like spending time with friends. I hope I have helped you see that healthy friendships are vital to stress-relief and your sense of well-being. Here are a few ways to fit more time with your BFF's in your busy schedule:

- **Don't do it alone.** We all have to eat, shop, and run errands. Why not call a friend and ask her to join you to run Saturday errands? You both probably have similar mundane things to get done. Put on your jeans, t-shirts, and comfy shoes and do them together. You'll knock out your "to do" list while having a great time together.

What about special projects you need to do around the house, like re-decorating, painting a room, or gardening? Ask a friend to come over to help and make it a fun experience with some good food, music, and lively atmosphere. Just be sure to return the favor when she calls.

In today's world, if you wait until you have leisure time to hang out with a friend, you may never get any. Reach out to that special pal and get things done together.

- **Use drive time.** The average American commute time to and from work is 46 minutes. Add the time we spend in our cars hauling children to and from activities and we practically live in our vehicles. Consider using your after work drive time to phone a good friend to chat. Chances are she's also driving home and it's a good time for her to connect. Use the drive time to chit chat, vent, or just catch up on the little things that make life worth living.

- **Schedule it.** According to Gallup research, women who have at least three or four good friends that they spend time with perform better at work and are healthier overall. To me, it's important enough to schedule the time if necessary. Make a date to spend some quality

> *Women who have at least three or four good friends that they spend time with perform better at work and are healthier overall.*

time with your girlfriends. For example, have a girlfriend's night in honor of each person's birthday; or plan an annual weekend getaway. The ideas are endless. The key is to realize how important good friendships are to your health and intentionally cultivate them.

I must say this . . .

Not all relationships are stress-relieving. Some are riddled with envy, disloyalty, and competition. These kinds of relationships are actually toxic and hazardous to your health. I encourage you to intentionally steer clear of "girlfriends" who present this kind of drama in your life. They are not your friends at all and you need to be honest with yourself about that. When it comes to friendship it's the quality, not the quantity, which matters most in our good health. A genuine friend is one who loves at all times—good and bad. Their loyalty has been tested over a period of time. They are treasures not quickly or easily found, but worth the effort. If you have just one girlfriend you trust who celebrates your successes and shares in your failures, you are rich. Hold on to her like she is a gift from God, because she is.

> *A genuine friend is one who loves at all times—good and bad.*

"A friend loves at all times, and a brother (sister) is born for adversity."

Proverbs 17:17

Right Now

Do you have friends who you genuinely love that you have lost contact with? Why?

When will you reach out to re-connect? How will you stay connected?

CONCLUSION

"There's a difference between interest and commitment. When you're interested in doing something, you do it only when circumstances permit. When you're committed to something, you accept no excuses, only results."

Anonymous

"Unless commitment is made, there are only promises and hopes; but no plans."

Peter F. Drucker

I asked a few friends to read through drafts of this book and one of them questioned if I should use the word "commitment" in the sub-title. She thought the term may be too strong for marketing purposes. It may intimidate potential readers because this generation steers clear of commitment. Maybe I should call the sub-title "5 Simple *Principles* That Can Save Your Life"? Of course, I want as many people to buy the book as possible, so I seriously considered her recommendation. I decided to stick with the word "commitment" and here is why.

Information and knowledge are good. But only that which you apply consistently will impact your life. Nothing in this book will help you if you don't do it. You must follow through. You must commit. The truth is that I would still be in the same stressed-out, unhealthy, and unhappy place if I had not committed to the principles I outline in this book. I don't just *know* them, but I actually *do* them consistently and intentionally. That is how my life was saved.

Wanting to live a longer, stronger life is the beginning. Unfortunately, desiring it is not enough. Having the knowledge is not enough either. Change requires commitment to a course of action. You will never see results in anything if you don't stick with a proven plan long enough for it to produce. Commitment is the key to any form of success in life.

Commitment is the act of pledging, involving, and engaging oneself. It begins with the powerful statement: "I will." "I will" is an emphatic declaration that carries a lot of weight. It means you are exerting your personal freedom and authority to choose your actions. The quality of your life is inextricably tied to your decisions—your will.

> *Commitment is the act of pledging, involving, and engaging oneself. It begins with the powerful statement: "I will."*

Let me ask you these questions: can you identify the sources of stress, tension, and burdens in your life? Do you acknowledge that if you don't combat them, they have the potential to create major health issues and even shorten your life? Do you want to live longer, stronger and more peacefully? Then you're going to have to consider a different lifestyle than you currently have. You will have to learn to respond differently to life's challenges. It will take courage and, yes, commitment to form a new set of healthier habits.

The path to a more peaceful way of life is not always easy to find in our success-driven culture. In some areas, you will have to live counter-culturally, resisting much of the "have-it—all" propaganda you hear. Trying to keep up with society's profit-driven expectations of you is exhausting. Give it up and embrace the wisdom of God for a healthier lifestyle and lasting success. Consider these words of Christ in Matthew 7:13,14:

> *"Enter by the narrow gate; for wide is the gate and broad is the way that leads to destruction, and there are many who go in by it. Because narrow is the gate and difficult is the way which leads to life, and there are few who find it."*

I am on a quest to stay in the way that leads to real life filled with significance and treasures that money cannot buy. Christ and his glorious wisdom is that Way. My prayer is that you and multitudes of others will join me.

Say this aloud with me: I want to live!

Many Blessings,

Genette

If you enjoyed *Fight Stress & Live: 5 Simple Commitments That Can Save Your Life*, Genette Howard is the ideal inspirational speaker for your next women's event!

In a world where sickness, stress and relational strife are the norm for women, Genette believes that you were created to rise above it and live an extraordinary life. Diseases don't have to be fatal. Relationships can mend. You can have profound joy and peace everyday. You just need the right information, inspiration, and motivation to begin to thrive.

That's what Genette Howard delivers in her dynamic, spiritually centered and information-packed messages and programs. She will leave you and your audience inspired, informed, and hungry for more of life. As a working wife and mother of six daughters, Genette is "every woman" and will quickly engage your group with her own stories of struggles, breakthroughs and strategies to thrive.

Genette's most requested topics include:

- Thrive! How to Win Over Stress and Love Your Life
- 5 Keys to Powerful Prayer
- The Wonder of a Woman
- How to Work Like a Woman
- 10 Things Every Woman Needs to Know About Men

If you would like to know more about booking Genette for a keynote, breakout, or workshop, please contact her at 479-251-7327. Or email questions to Genette@GenetteHoward.com

Share this book!

Quantity discounts are available. Please contact us for a quote. We also have personalized, autographed copies available.